Get Rightsized

With the Dish Diet™

Danuta Highet, BSME & MM

Published By Maidin Works
2020

Published by:
MW Maidin Works, P.O. Box 910, New Smyrna Beach, FL 32170
www.MaidinWorks.com.

The publisher may produce the book in all formats (electronic, audio and print) where some content available in print may not be available in electronic or audio books, and vice versa.

Photos and images by Adobe.com and Peter Nguyen
Cover, Book Layout and Grizmo® designed by Peter Nguyen
Grizmo® name and image are registered trademarks of Foqus, Inc.

Trademarks and Service-marks TM & SM: Dish Diet™, Dish Size™, Bite Size™, CDM - Caloric Density Mark™ and Get Rightsized™, and US10311748B2 and US20120077154A1 patents are exclusive property of Foqus, Inc. and can only be used under the licenses granted by Foqus, Inc.

Printed in the United States of America.

Table of Contents

Preface

I am not trying to sell you a diet or a set of dishes. I am trying to sell you the idea that you can easily implement today and reap the benefits in your health and well-being tomorrow.

This is not the same old diet book. There are no recipes to follow, no meals to buy, no measuring or weighing food, no calculating calories. This book will help you change your life through small, gradual changes. You have all the power you need to change your life.

Ever since I can remember I was uncertain about how much food I should serve myself. When I had my children, the dilemma switched to them. When my daughter Katherine (who has autism) became a teenager, she could not decide how much to serve herself. She started to gain weight. What should have been a joyful time became a battle ground with tears and disappointments. I was fighting my own battle with weight gain and had difficulty maintaining a healthy weight.

I became passionate about solving this problem. I knew there had to be a simple way to control your portion that even a child could implement. Thus I got the idea of The Dish Diet.

Whether you consider yourself in perfect shape or are struggling with maintaining an ideal weight, you can benefit from reading this book. It will help simplify and manage daily food consumption and allows you to gradually achieve your health goals. It's time to stop thinking about tallying calories and planning every bite.

Chances are that you already have all the tools you need to lose weight and maintain a healthy weight. Using your existing everyday dishware, you can slowly rightsize your food intake and lose weight at your own pace. The Dish Diet's Patented[1] method will free your mind from the worry surrounding food. It's time to enjoy your life without guilt. No more measuring or counting. You can eat your way into a healthy lifestyle. Permanently.

Every person big or small has the rightsized, healthy portion size for them for every stage of their life. I have patented a methodology for a new way of eating. It's portion control on auto-pilot. It works and is so easy.

Let's "Get Rightsized"!

Postscript

"Today is the first day of the rest of your life." [2]

CHARLES DEDERICH

Many diets ask you to spend a lot of money on special food or meetings. They ask you to invest hours of your time in planning your meals counting calories and exercise. All I ask is that you read this book. What do you have to lose?

Chapter 1

Imagine

*"The courage to imagine
the otherwise is our greatest resource,
adding color and suspense to all our life."* [3]

DANIEL J. BOORSTIN

You wake up in the morning and are ready to start the day. You take a quick shower and make your breakfast. You go to your cupboard, pick a bowl size 6 and fill it up. You pack your lunch in a size 6 container and head off to work.

After work you head to a Bistro. You feel like having a sweet drink, so you order it two sizes smaller to stick to your personalized meal size. You ask for a soup and select your dish size and spoon size. The server happily obliges.

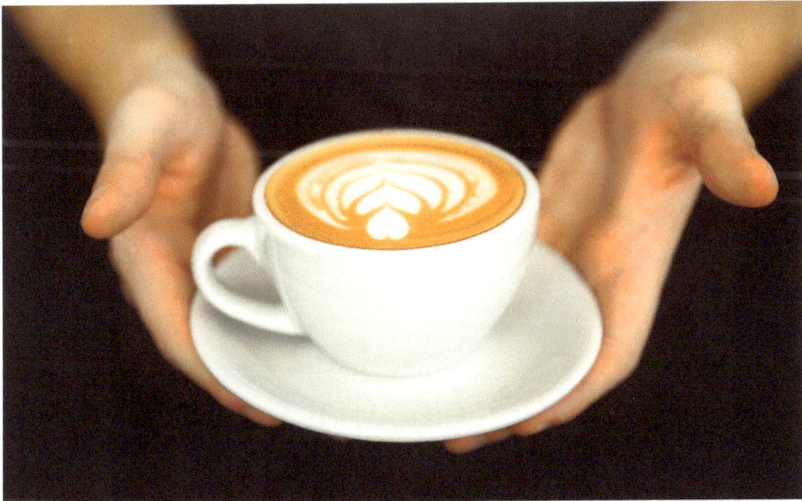

On your way home, you hit the supermarket. You need to pick up some frozen meals because you will have a busy week. The packages are clearly identified with your meal size, making it easy and stress-free to select your favorites.

You can cook next week, so you look at your app and search your favorite recipes by simply picking the meal size you want. The app provides a list of how much of each ingredient you need. You bring your food home and put it away. The rest of the night belongs to you.

Can you envision our future like this? You know the right meal size to maintain a healthy lifestyle and focus on life's most enjoyable activities. You can go anywhere and get the Rightsized meal portion every time to establish a healthy way of eating. The term "diet" can reclaim it's original meaning: the food you eat.

Imagine a world without sizes. You walk into the shoe store and your salesperson brings you the biggest shoe that it carries. You try to buy a shirt and a clerk hands you a one-size-fit-all tall. Today, you can ask for a ring by size but you can't buy a meal in the size that's Rightsized for you. It's one-size-fits-all.

What if you could optimize your meal size to where you can just serve and eat and not worry if you will gain weight? Every dish, bowl, cup, spoon and fork has a size, so you can stick to your Rightsized portion at every meal. Imagine that every spoon you pick up has a size listed on it. Every plate or bowl or cup or glass has a size marked. All you will need is to pick your sized dishware and utensils, fill it, eat, and stay healthy.

Imagine that...

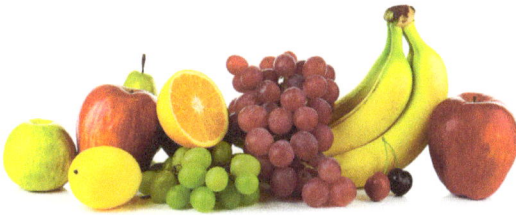

Food for thought	
Portion	Portions have sizes.
Dishware	Dishware has sizes.
Utensils	Utensils have sizes.
Imagine	A world where all the eating-ware has size that helps you auto-rightsize all of your meals...

Chapter 2

Illusion is Real

*"Perceive that
which cannot be seen with the eye."* [4]

MIYAMOTO MUSASHI

When we were children, we watched illusionists and magicians perform tricks in front of our eyes. We believed in magic. As adults we know that the secret to magic is knowing how to do the trick.

We don't believe that we could be misled by illusions, yet every day we are. Only now its called "marketing" or "advertising". Companies use many proven techniques to get us to buy more and eat more food.

Our eyes don't communicate perfectly with our brain so we miss important information. It has to do with the position of our eyes and the delay in processing sight information. This focal arrangement allows us to see depth (three-dimensional objects), but we also can be tricked by illusions.

Look at the white dots in the diagram below. Your eyes will make you think that the small dots are bouncing from black to white.

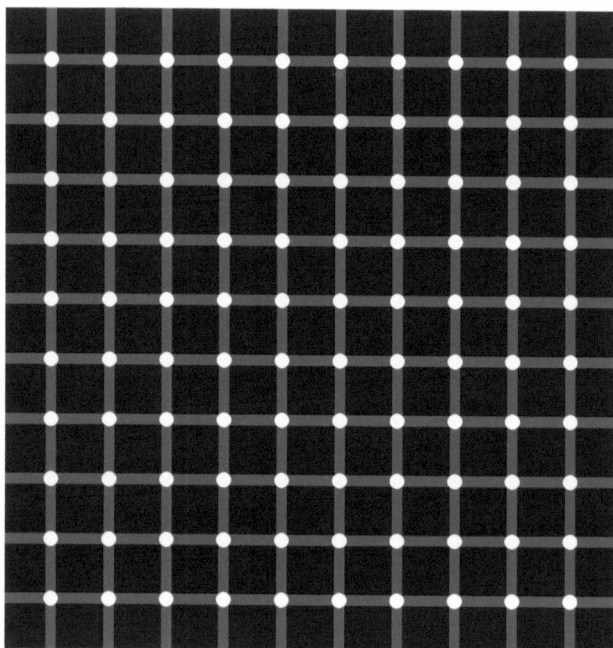

A similar illusion occurs when you see the circles on the next page. As the black circles get bigger, the white circles appear to get smaller. They only appear smaller. Every white circle is the exact same size.

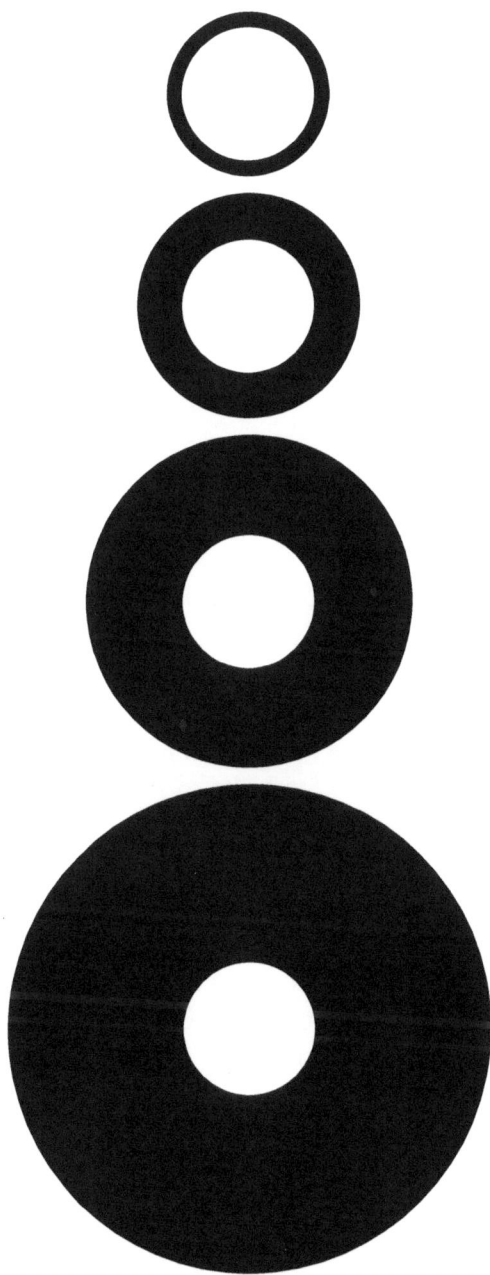

Visual illusion by **JOSEPH DELBOEUF**

Remember when new dishware arrived in stores? We thought, "Wow, food will look so elegant on the new bigger plates." They showed up in beautiful designs and the size of a platter. The most chic restaurants use the biggest plates.

Over the last 30 to 40 years dishes have been growing. A typical dinner plate used to be 9 inches across, now it is 11 to 12 inches or more in diameter. Some restaurants use 16 to 17 inch plates. What's wrong with this? We did not realize that our food appeared smaller. So now with the big plate, not only do we have more room on our plate for more food, our eyes want to fill the space so it appears the same as it did before.

Let's say your previous dinner plate was 9 inches in diameter and typically you left about 2 inches from the edge when you served yourself. When you switched to an 11 inch diameter plate you will up-size your portion until it leaves about 2 inches around your plate. Now you added a lot more food.

The same optical illusion you see with the white circles affects how we view our food. As our dishware got bigger we had to fill up our plates with more food just to feel like we are eating the same amount.

On the next page, you see a single serving on a plate. Watch what happens to the serving as it is placed on the next larger size plate. The serving appears to be shrinking. When you keep increasing the plate size, your brain believes there is less and less food. By the time it's on the big plate, the serving looks like a snack.

As the plates got bigger, other table accessories grew too. When the bowls got bigger, the quantity of food delivery increased even more than with the plates.

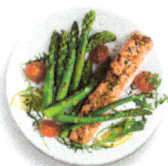

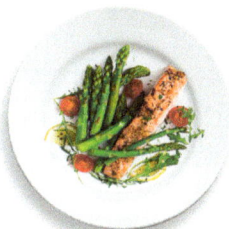

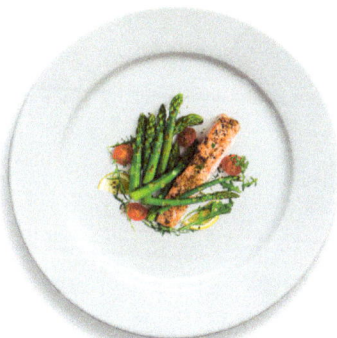

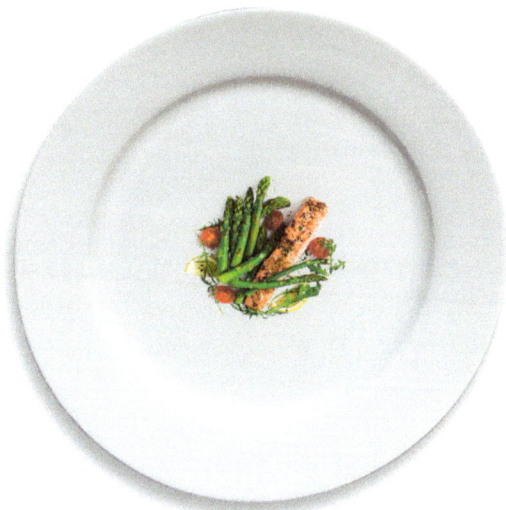

Even though the plates grew just a couple of inches in diameters, volumetrically the bowls increased in size at a higher rate. Now, to match these larger plates, all other eating-ware had to be up-sized. Spoons got bigger, so did the forks, cups, and glasses. "Supersized" plates are now the "norm" everywhere.

THE SUPERSIZED DISHWARE
MADE OUR FOOD APPEAR SMALLER.

To keep up with the growing size of plates, we put more food on the plates than ever before. Thus, we ate more, drank more, and still felt hungry. Deceived by the larger dishware, we think we need more food.

So everything had to grow just to make us feel like we were eating the same amount. Restaurants increased the amount of food they serve. Pizzas grew, bagels grew, bread slices grew, soda, chocolates, even fresh strawberries.

We started to reach for the bigger spoon and the bigger fork. Now, not only did we eat more food, we placed more food into every bite. We transferred more food from the plate to our mouths at a faster rate.

Our brains are not paying any attention. We used to eat a bowl of cereal with a teaspoon. Now that "teaspoon" is the size of a soup spoon. When we ate our cereal with the smaller teaspoon it took us 40 spoonfuls to finish. Now with the larger spoon it may take 20 spoonfuls.

The brain doesn't consider what spoon was used. All it knows is we took only 20 spoonfuls when we used to get 40. Now we feel hungry.

When our cups and glasses got bigger they impacted our weight as well. If you just drank water it would not matter, but soda and sugar/corn syrup-loaded juices just add more pounds to our bodies without any additional satisfaction.

When we use a big plate or drink from a bigger glass, we consume more food. When we eat with bigger utensils, we eat more food per bite.

Some of today's cereal and soup bowls can hold a quart (32 oz), of food. When we put a 3/4 cup (6 oz) serving inside a quart-sized bowl, that bowl looks almost empty.

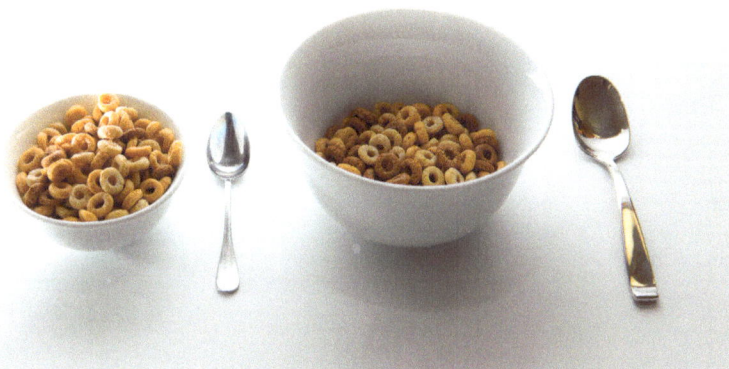

The typical recommended serving size on many cereal boxes is about 3/4 cup to 1 cup, yet the picture on the box shows a much bigger bowl and a much bigger portion than the recommended serving size.

So we justify pouring four, five or more servings thinking "the serving size" is for children, that the recommended portion can't really be for an adult. Yet, the serving size listed on the label **is** for an adult. That is all our bodies need.

Pizza example: As Pizza expanded in diameter from 10" to 17" or even bigger, each slice grew in multiples.

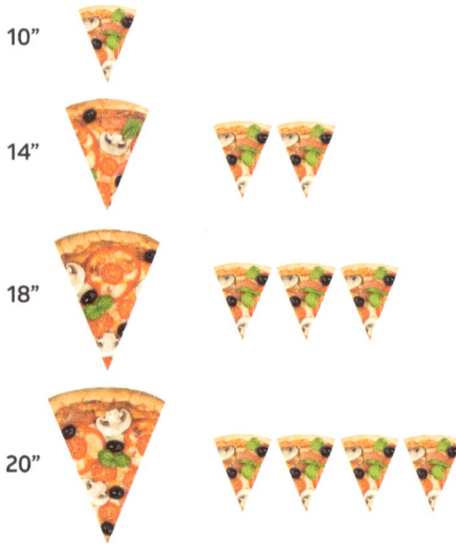

Pizza diameter in	Area of a slice in^2	Percent bigger than 10" pie slice	
10"	10		—
11"	12		21 %
12"	14		44 %
13"	17		69 %
14"	19		96 %
15"	22		125 %
16"	25		156 %
17"	28		189 %
18"	32		224 %
19"	35		261 %
20"	39		300 %

This shows you that the 20-inch pizza pie single slice equates to 4 slices of the 10-inch pizza which means four times more calories per slice. That's one slice of the supersized pie is now 1/2 the pie. Shrink the diameter of the pizza you are buying and ask them to "double slice" it. You will feel more satisfied and shrink your portion as well.

ALL the dishes, and ALL our food has expanded in size since the 1980's. The plates, the cups, the bowls, the snack bowls, the wine glasses, the burgers, the fries, the bagels... they all have been SUPERSIZED. As a result, we are becoming SUPERSIZED, too.

*"If you want to be right-sized in body,
you've got to get rid of the supersize way of life."* [5]

BOB HARPER

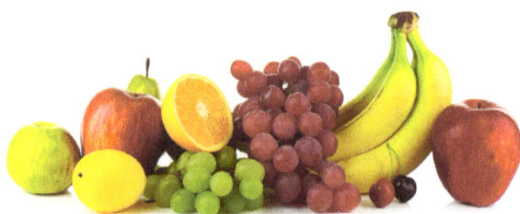

Food for thought	
Dishware	Dishware expanded in size.
Portions	Portions grew with the dishware.
Bodies	Bodies got supersized with supersized portions and dishware.
Dishware	Change your dishware!

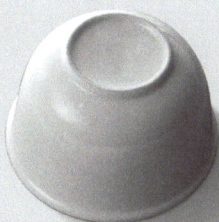

Bowl	Weight management tool

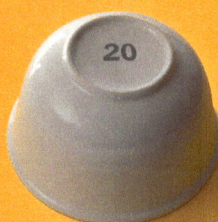

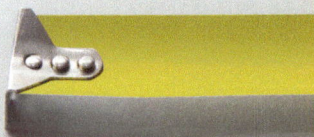

Tape	Measuring Tool

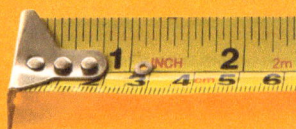

Chapter 3

What is the Dish Diet?

*"A person with a new idea
is a crank until the idea succeeds."* [6]

MARK TWAIN

Many diets look at the total caloric value of your daily food consumption and try to cut it down drastically. If you do this, initially it will be exciting and motivating. You will lose lots of pounds quickly. But your body will start to lower your burn rate and you will lose less and less as weeks go by.

Controlling your portion size is the most effective and successful way to lose weight in the long run. Until now there was no practical way to size your portion. The Dish Diet gives you control when you have the highest power of control, before you start to eat the first bite.

You don't have to focus on counting points or calories. You don't have to eat expensive, tasteless prepackaged foods. You don't have to attend meetings. You can lose weight as fast or as slowly as you want.

The Dish Diet is different because it works with your body and brain to help you succeed. It helps you eat fewer calories over time without suddenly starving yourself. Research shows that we can easily eat 100 to 200 calories more or less each day without your body noticing[7]. With The Dish Diet you will lower the average daily calorie consumption a little at a time.

The Dish Diet looks at the volumetric amount of food we eat and not the calories. You will not see any recipes or directions of what to eat and what not to eat. It focuses on helping you to change the volumetric amount of food you eat.

Why volumetrically? Because you can use the same illusion that got you to where you are today to fight the illusion in reverse. The Dish Diet helps you shrink your portion size. It will help your brain to learn what is the rightsized portion for you.

Just as an example, let's say that every day you consume a 1/2 gallon of food and drink. That is 64 ounces of each. A typical diet might tell you cut this in half. Of course you will lose weight quickly initially, but you will feel so deprived that at some point you will quit.

But what if you went down an ounce in one week? Do you think you would notice? And if you did this every two weeks, in 64 weeks (a little over a year) you would gradually (without deprivation) cut your daily portion in half by reducing your daily portion by an ounce every two weeks. The difference is that since you arrived there gradually, you have retrained your brain to realize that this is the rightsized portion for you. It will be your new normal.

The Dish Diet looks at the eating process as a whole and focuses on the volumetric amount of food we eat and how we eat, not just calories. It introduces four new concepts :

- **Portion Size**™
- **Dish Size**™
- **Bite Size**™
- **CDM - Caloric Density Mark**™

The Portion Size and Dish Size have the biggest impact in helping you manage your weight. The Bite Size will help you succeed by changing how fast you eat so that you feel more fulfilled with every meal. The CDM will make it easier to make healthier food choices.

What is Portion Size ?

If you look at the following chart, it shows how the Portion Size gradually decreases in volume with each size from 31 to 0. The bottom color of the column represents a volume of the portion size. The top color represents the "Extra" portion that makes it to the next size. 0-Portion Size is just the orange bottom portion of 1-Portion Size. The patented Dish Diet Sizing System works in a way that every "Extra" gets a little smaller as sizes go down.

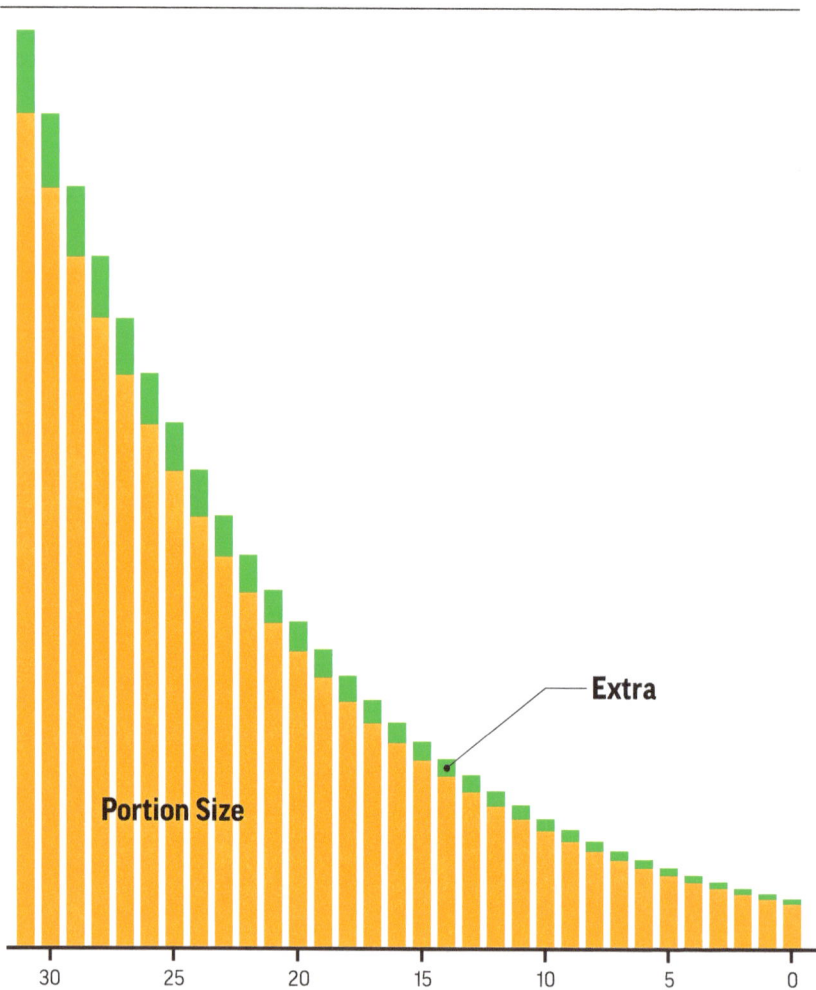

As you go down in Portion Size the "hump" of reducing the portion gets smaller. This keeps you motivated to go down in size until you get to your "Rightsize".

The Portion Size assigns a numerical value to a volume of food. The Dish Size assigns the same (equivalent) numerical value to eatingware that just fits the Portion Size. I will use a malleable flexible character who I named Grizmo® to help me demonstrate how the sizing process works. Grizmo® represents the volumetric amount of food for a given Portion Size.

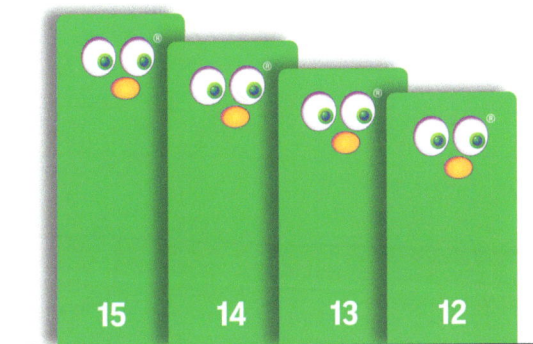

Grizmo® has the ability to volumetrically adjust to the size we need by climbing into all types of containers and tell us the container Dish Size. The Dish Size can be assigned to every type of dish, box, plate or cup and even a flat surface.

The two drawings below show how Grizmo® fits into containers to give it a size. The first image represents a Grizmo® Portion Size 32. The second shows how he fits inside a container. If you notice his "head" is sticking out above the container to account for food served above the rim. The third picture shows an empty container that now has an established Dish Size 32. The same measuring process is used for every dish, plate, bowl, or container.

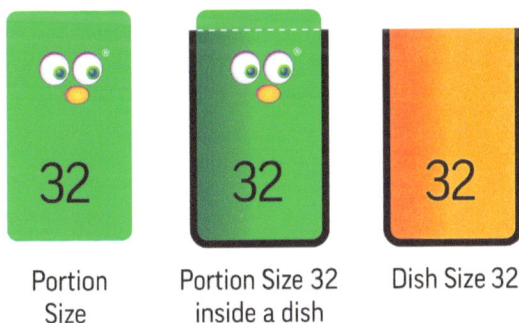

| Portion Size | Portion Size 32 inside a dish | Dish Size 32 |

Portion Size	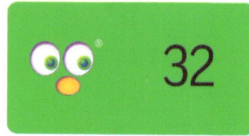
Portion Size 32 inside a dish	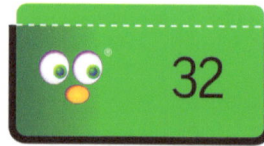
Dish Size 32	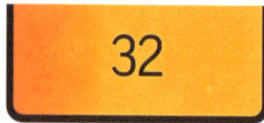

No matter the shape, Grizmo® can climb in and tell you what Portion Size will fit in your dish. Once Grizmo® fits just right, it will tell you what is the Dish Size of that container.

All you need to know is your Dish Size to stick to your Portion Size without having to check the volume ever again.

Think of the Dish Size like a set of wrenches for your meal. When you need to tighten a nut all you need to know is the nut size. Then you pick the right size wrench to tighten it. Same goes for your Dish Size. Once you know the size of your dish, you select it, fill it and eat and you can stick to your Rightsized Portion no matter what type of container it is or what type of food you eat.

SIMILARLY DIMENSIONED DISHWARE
ARE NOT CREATED EQUAL.

If you compare one plate that is 11 inches wide vs another of the same width you will find that they hold different amounts of food. While doing research on sizing of dishware, I called one of the United States' largest dishware manufacturers and asked for technical support. A very cordial tech support person listened as I explained that I needed the dimensions of their dishware.

"Madam, all the dimensions are available on our website."

"I found the volume of the bowls," I said, *"but I couldn't find the volume of the plates. Do you have the volume of your plates?"* The line went silent. I thought I lost the connection. *"Are you there?"*

Another long pause preceded an incredulous, sarcastic response: *"Madam, ... plates don't have volume!?!"*

"Yes they do," I said and I tried to explain further. Realizing that I was not going to get the information, I thanked her and moved onto measuring the dishware myself.

Yes, plates have volume, lots of volume.

Look at a cross-section of a plate. The basic design of any plate is concave. In essence, it facilitates eating just like a shallow bowl. We judge the total quantity of food we serve ourselves based on what we see on top. What's underneath is hidden from us to judge.

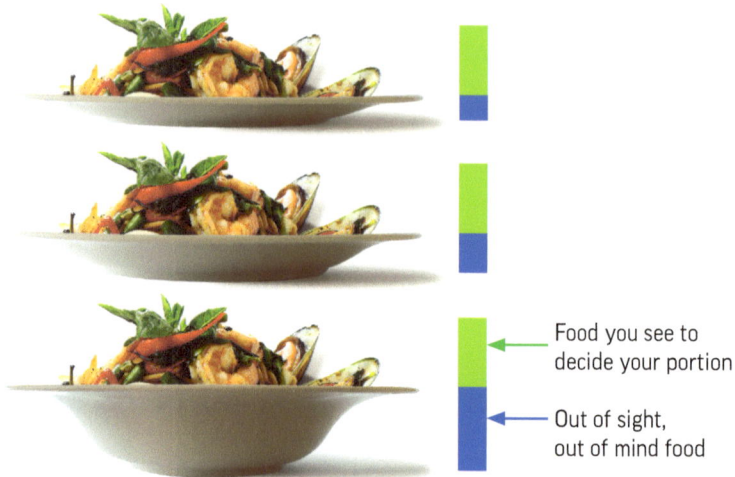

Food you see to decide your portion

Out of sight, out of mind food

The picture shows three different styles of plates showing the same amount of the visible food above the plate. The only plate lacking volume inside is one that is completely flat. The deeper the plate the more it acts like a bowl and will contain additional volume. Bowls hide much more food than plates.

Some plates I have measured contained 32 ounces of food inside the plate — that's four cups of food that your eye does not see. Plates that look similar can deliver different portions. Size all the plates you use.

You are retraining your brain and your thoughts to eat the Rightsized portion for you. The number of calories always fluctuates, but in the long run they average out.

What is a Bite Size?

The Dish Diet goes beyond any other diet in another way. It addresses how fast you eat with the Bite Size. As the dishware got bigger the utensils got bigger. Similar to the Portion Size, the patented volumetric portion of food that you put in your mouth with a spoon or a fork is represented by Bite Size.

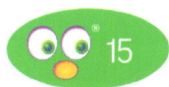

Bite Size 15 of food

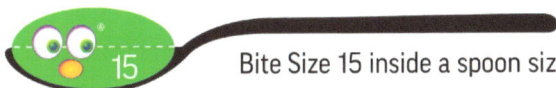

Bite Size 15 inside a spoon size 15

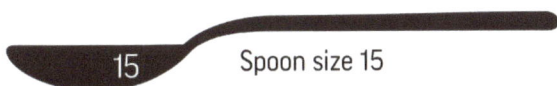

Spoon size 15

As Grizmo® sits comfortably in a spoon or a fork it gives that utensil it's Bite Size. The smaller your fork or spoon the less food you can load up on it with every bite. The smaller the Bite Size the more time it will take to finish the meal, and the more satisfied you will feel.

The Bite Size controls how fast you eat while the Dish Size controls the total amount you eat. You are in control of both.

What is Caloric Density Mark (CDM)?

As you start using the Dish Diet – depending how healthy your typical diet is – your Dish Size may get so small that you will feel deprived. The Dish Diet introduces another new concept: Caloric Density Mark (CDM). This is a way to quickly express how many calories are in a volume of food. So if you have an ounce (volume) of cheese or an ounce (volume) of milk they will have a different CDM.

Do calories matter? Of course they do.
But our brain does not perceive or taste the number of calories.

35

The Caloric Density Mark uses letters to indicate how calorie dense the foods are. The closer to the beginning of alphabet the lower the number of calories in the same volume of food.

When you are ready to change what you eat you can look at the CDM of your typical diet and by shifting some or all of your diet to lower your CDM your Rightsized Portion Size may actually increase in size. (I will explain this further in Chapter 5).

Reducing the Portion Size/Dish Size/Bite Size in small size increments will not make you feel deprived. Your dishware and utensils will get a little smaller with each incremental adjustment, but because of the illusion, your food will appear a little bigger. You will fill up your plate with less food but you will feel like you are eating the same amount as before. You end up eating less, yet feeling satisfied.

With the Dish Diet, you're not just shrinking your plate, you are shrinking your thoughts too. You are gradually finding out what is the right Portion Size for you so that **you** can get **Rightsized**.

*"This is one small step for [a] man,
one giant leap for mankind."* [8]

NEIL ARMSTRONG

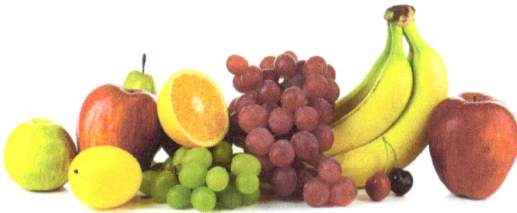

Food for thought	
Illusion	1. Illusion is Real. 2. Food appears larger on smaller plate. 3. Fight illusion with illusion.
Portion Size	Knowing your Portion Size puts you in control of your portions.
Dish Size	Makes portion control easy.
Adjust	Adjust your Portion/Dishware Size up or down as your lifestyle and diet changes.
Bite Size	Slows down your eating so that you enjoy food longer and feel more fulfilled.
Smaller	Smaller dishware will make you think you are eating more while you are eating less and feel more satisfied.

Plate	Weight management tool

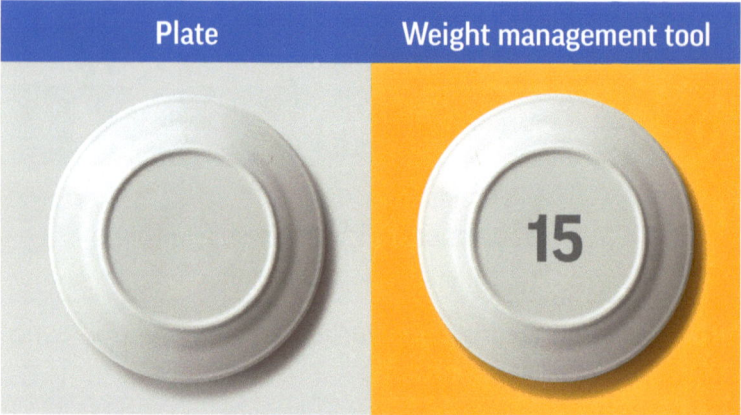

Heavy object	Exercise Tool

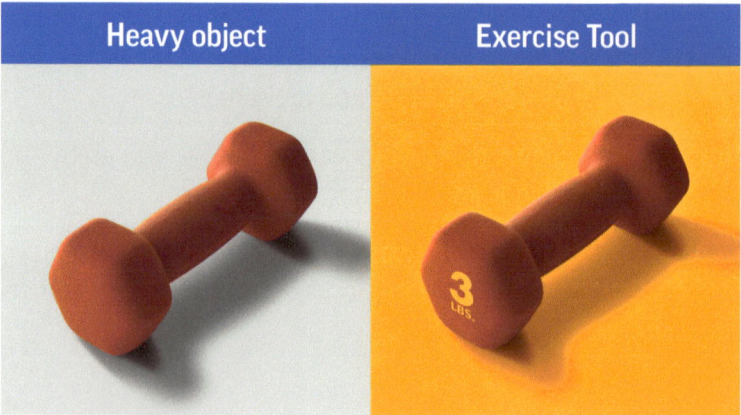

Chapter 4

How do I start?

*"A man may die, nations may rise and fall,
but an idea lives on."* [9]

JOHN F. KENNEDY

To start the Dish Diet is easy. You do not necessarily need to purchase the set of dishes offered on DishDiet.com. You can put a nail in a wall with a brick, yet a hammer makes it easier.

Until my mission is complete and all the dishware is identified with the Dish Diet Size, you can get a set of the Dish Diet dishes or you can use Grizmo® to help size your own dishes.

**CHECK WITH YOUR DOCTOR BEFORE TRYING
ANY NEW DIET OR WEIGHT LOSS PLAN**

You do not need to purchase anything more than this book to get started. The Dish Diet consists of four simple steps:

STEP 1 - Figure out your Dish Diet Size
STEP 2 - Fill your dish with food and eat
STEP 3 - Check if gaining, losing, or maintaining weight
STEP 4 - Adjust your dish size based on trends in Step 3

STEP 1: Figure out your Dish Diet Size

All you need to size your dishware is a measuring cup and a ruler. Fill your dish with water all the way to the rim and record how many ounces of water fit inside your dish. Take a ruler and measure how wide your dish is across the center of it. These two numbers are all you need to fill the form on the DishSize.com website to size your dish.

**GO TO DISHSIZE.COM WEBSITE
TO SIZE YOUR OWN DISHWARE.**

STEP 2: Serve food and eat

You need to refuel every three-to-four hours, pick the dish that's your size, and fill it up. You will not need to think about how many calories are in the chicken, the potato, the broccoli, or the carrots. The number of calories may vary per meal just like the amount of activity you will do from day to day. As long as you stick to the same Dish Size, you will consume an average daily amount.

You can lose weight while eating the foods you love. You do not need to buy expensive diet foods. There is nothing special or magical about these foods. The diet foods contain the same ingredients that you use. Most of them are one-size-fit-all. You can implement the right-size-for-you with your own dishware.

STEP 3: Check if gaining, losing, or maintaining weight

Weigh yourself every day, at the same time each day. The best time may be each morning before breakfast and before you take a shower, so that your weight is at its lowest.

This weight will vary if you eat late at night. After a week of using The Dish Diet dishes for all your meals, check if your weight is changing.

Because your weight will vary daily, you can detect trends easier if you average out your weight in pounds each week:

Week 1:
174, 170, 173, 172, 171, 173, 173 Average daily: 172 pounds

Week 2:
172, 172, 171, 173, 170, 171, 170 Average daily: 171 pounds

Week 3:
170, 171, 168, 169, 167, 168, 170 Average daily: 169 pounds

This shows a weight loss of one pound from Week 1 to Week 2 and further weight loss of about two pounds the following week.

STEP 4: Adjust your Dish Size based on your weight loss trend in Step 3

To decide what to do the next week, follow these simple directions below unless your doctor gives you other guidelines. Most doctors recommend a maximum weight loss of 2 pounds per week for an adult. If you are very overweight your doctor may recommend reducing your size quicker or in bigger increments.

DIRECTIONS (FOR ADULTS ONLY)

If you:

- Lost three or more pounds, the plate /bowl is too small. Change to the next larger Dish Size.

- Lost one or two pounds, great. That's a recommended rate for adult weight loss. Are you feeling OK? If everything is going well, continue using the same Dish Size.

- No change, then you are still eating too much. Lower your Dish Size.

- Gained weight. The dishware you used before you started was causing you to keep gaining weight. That's why you probably were constantly Yo-Yo dieting. You may be reducing the rate you are gaining at first. Simply adjust until you find the Right-sized Dish Size where you start to lose weight.

**Dishware got so big that you may need to
go down many sizes just to start losing weight.**

How fast you lose weight is up to you. You can drastically reduce your Portion Size by skipping multiple sizes. Your Doctor can help you make that decision, but drastically reducing your portion size to quickly lose weight will lead to the feeling of deprivation. At some point you are likely to revert to old habits.

Slow and steady is healthier and easier, since it maximizes your metabolic rate! The Rightsized Dish Size will depend on how quickly you want to lose weight and how deprived you will feel if you go down in size too quickly. It's not just your stomach that needs to shrink, it's your thoughts. You need to unlearn what's become habit.

You will be amazed how little food you need to refuel.

The Dish Diet is about optimizing your portions to fit your "portionality" so you can eat on autopilot. You could adjust all dishware by one Dish Size down or chose one dish at a time.

Type of Dishware	Starting Dish Size	Week 1 Dish Size	Week 2 Dish Size
Dinner plate	28	27	26
Dinner bowl	28	27	26
Salad Plate	18	17	16
Saucer	10	10	10
Mug	16	15	14
Glass	15	14	13
Water glass	15	18	19
Wine glass	12	11	10
Snack dish	16	15	14
Snack bag	12	11	10

The more you transition to one size for all your meals the quicker your brain will learn your Rightsized Dish Size. If you shrink your dishes but don't shrink your utensils, you will feel deprived. Changing the size of your place setting will help you succeed.

Use illusion to fight illusion.

The illusion that got you to where you are today can take you to the right path. The brain can reverse the ruse in your favor. Simply, shrink your dishware size slowly and gradually. The food will appear bigger so you will need less yet feel just as full. It works!

If you want to lose weight, but measuring dishware seems to complex, and you can't afford the Dish Diet Dishware – simply shrink the dishes you currently use. The portion size will not be as gradual and you may feel a little more deprived but eventually you will find the dish that works for you. Make your salad plate your dinner plate, your butter plate your lunch plate, etc.

Reducing the dishware size that holds the largest portions like a dinner plate, and highest in calories like a desert plate, snack containers, and high calorie drinks will give you the quickest results. At first glance it seems like a lot to do. It's not.

Once you conquer your meal dishware for dinner, lunch, and breakfast expand the Dish Diet concept to other aspects of eating. You can measure each dish in minutes. Once you do, you are free to enjoy your life.

Rightsize your drink-ware: Our environment has added a lot of high-caloric density foods in the form of liquids. A milkshake is a huge meal, not an addition to a meal. A typical large chocolate milkshake can have 1300 calories. For some of us, that is more food than we need for a day.

SOME RESTAURANTS CALL A MILKSHAKE "SNACK-SIZED" AND IT HAS 420 CALORIES.

Sodas, juices, alcohol, and many cafe drinks are very high in calories. All drink-ware has exploded in size and now delivers bigger portion size. Reducing the size of high-calorie drinks is a quick way to lower your daily Portion Size. Just like you measure your dishware you can measure your drink-ware on DishSize.com.

Rightsize your snack-ware: What if your Portion Size gets sooooo small and you are still not losing weight?

This can happen when you are consuming too many calories just in snack food and drinks. A snack is a tease for your brain. It's usually food high in sugar and rich in calories that are concentrated in a small portion.

If you do snack, you can use the The Dish Diet Size to Rightsize your snack size as well. Use the The Dish Diet Rightsized dishes for snacks. Decrease the size of your snack dish, just like you decrease the size of the dish for your main meals.

You may find that splitting the meal into two smaller portions and eating the second half instead of a snack will keep you satiated longer than a bigger meal plus a snack.

Rightsize your silverware: Utensils control how fast we eat and how much food we transfer per bite. Now when you select your spoon or your fork you will control how fast you eat. The bigger the Bite Size, the faster you will load your mouth without feeling satiated. The more food you have in your mouth, the less chance your palate has to taste every morsel and communicate that information to your brain.

Rightsize your diet ware: We all have our own best way to lose weight. If you feel that you need a commercial diet to help you, the Dish Diet will complement any other diet.

If you use a diet that sends you entrees in the mail, just transfer that entree to the dish that just fits it. Then measure that dish and you can transition to that Dish Size.

It doesn't matter how you get to the Rightsized portion as long as you do. Some of you may implement the Dish Diet going one size at a time and it might take you months or years to get you to the Rightsized you. In this case it's not the journey, it's the destination.

"I've missed more than 9,000 shots in my career.
I've lost almost 300 games. Twenty-six times,
I've been trusted to take the game-winning shot and missed.
I've failed over and over again in my life.
And that is why I succeed." [10]

MICHAEL JORDAN

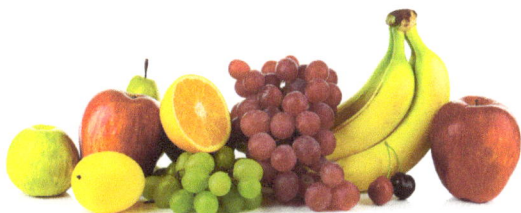

Food for thought	
Lose	Lose weight by adjusting your Dish Size gradually at your own pace.
Gain	Gain confidence that you can control your weight no matter what life may bring.
Easy	Losing weight can be easy when you have the right tools.
Tools	Your tools are in your cabinets. Finding the Dish Diet Size once is a lot easier than measuring how many calories are in every meal
Change	Change how you eat so you can change how you live.

Chapter 5

Get Rightsized

*"A journey of a thousand miles
begins with a single step."* [11]

CONFUCIUS

Rightsized you, is **you** at the optimum healthy weight so you can do what you love to do. It's the weight where you are the strongest and fastest that you can be. This is the weight where your heart, your joints and all your organs think you are beautiful because their job just got so much easier. They don't need to struggle anymore.

Rightsized you can dance and run without feeling exhausted. Rightsized you can golf or play ball with your friends instead of watching it on TV. The kid in you wants to be Rightsized. You can get there again.

Once you succeed in making small, gradual changes in your eating, you can apply the same process to your life. There are simple measures you can take in your daily routine that will maximize your success and help you achieve the Rightsized healthy you.

Rightsize your meals

Think about how you get from the time you think about food to the point where you are finished eating. There are many steps that you can adjust through small changes that will help you succeed at home, at work, and at play.

When eating at home, you can serve yourself in the kitchen and put the leftovers away immediately. Have you ever thought to yourself after the first bite "Wow, I didn't realize how hungry I was!" Once you taste your first bite, it's difficult to stop eating.

You can eat everything you like, but if you eat foods that have high CDM, you will consume more calories per the same size portion. You can reduce your calorie consumption gradually by changing the CDM of the food you put on your plate.

Here is an example of the Caloric Density Mark, or CDM:

Carrots **A**
Cookies **F**
Cheese **M**

The lower the alphabet letter of the food the more of them you can eat. So, for example, ten cookies that have the CDM **A** will have the same number of calories as a single, same size cookie that has a CDM **J**. A child will be able to decide which snack bar is better for them, **A** or **J**, without having an understanding of calories.

Filling your dish with foods that have a CDM in the beginning of the alphabet will help you succeed in your quest for a healthy weight. Go to DishDiet.com to find the CDM for many foods.

Rightsize your restaurant experience

Try to order one course at a time. It will mean more work for the waiter and the kitchen but you can reward them with a higher tip.

Use the same Dish Diet Size you use at home. Ask for a box-to-go and pack the rest away before you start eating.

Knowing the portion you have is Rightsized before you taste the food is a huge help. Once the food is packed away and out of sight, you won't have "just one more bite." Chances are that by the time you get home, your stomach and your brain will both be satisfied.

Rightsize your family

"All great change in America begins at the dinner table." [12]

RONALD REAGAN

Parents generally instill lifelong habits in their children that will last throughout their lives. This means good habits or bad habits. Now parents have a tool to help their children eat the right amount of food every time.

**CONSULT WITH YOUR FAMILY DOCTOR
BEFORE CONSIDERING ANY DIET.**

The Dish Diet makes it easy for the whole family to get Rightsized and stay healthy. Every family member has their own weight considerations and their own distinctive metabolism.

Everyone has their own weight goals. Each member of your family can enjoy the same meal from a personalized Rightsized Dish. The family can be together without anyone feeling deprived. You might say, "This is changing how we used to eat." And you are right, but the environment has changed – and this simple change can make a difference for your family.

You will build healthy habits for life and give your children tools they can use in the future to stay healthy and Get Rightsized.

Rightsize your environment

Surroundings and how you live affect how much you eat. It is harder for you to lose weight when your world constantly reminds you of food. You can't eliminate your thoughts, but you can use your own marketing strategy to crave healthier food choices and healthier activities.

Making small changes in your surroundings at home and work (and even with friends) can help you make positive changes in your life. Look at where you work, where you live, where you spend your leisure time.

Are there any "food-thought" triggers? How much time do you spend in your kitchen? Fight marketing with marketing. What will make you think about walking, dancing, or playing sports? Surround yourself with positive visual reminders.

MARKETING WORKS.
MAKE IT WORK FOR YOU.

Rightsize your social events

Eating out with friends is tough when you are trying to lose weight. You can take simple steps to succeed outside your home environment.

If you meet in a restaurant, you can go to one with healthy choices. You can ask for a smaller dish and transfer the food you plan to eat and pack the rest to go. You can put something else in your hand to keep your hands occupied while you talk. Place the water glass next to your martini glass to give you a calorie-free alternative between sips. (See Appendix for more tips to Get Rightsized.)

The ideas presented in this book are simple solutions to a very complex problem. It's so much easier to gain weight than to lose weight. But I'll ask you again: What do you have to lose?

Imagine...Believe...

"Believe you can and you're halfway there." [13]

THEODORE ROOSEVELT

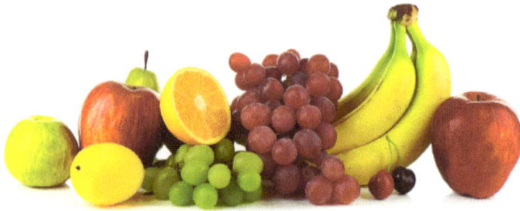

Food for thought	
Rightsize	Rightsize your eatingware to Rightsize your body.
Children	Learn to eat the Rightsized portion if they know their Dish Size.
Parents	Help set children's habits for a lifetime. Make those good habits.
Families	Families can help each other succeed in achieving health goals.
Home	Change your home to inspire you to a healthy and active lifestyle.
Work	Change your work surroundings to reflect success in every way throughout each day.

Get Rightsized - Rightsize Your Life

Mug	Weight management tool
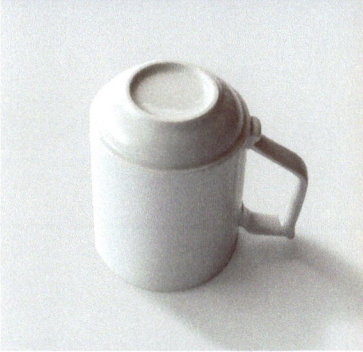	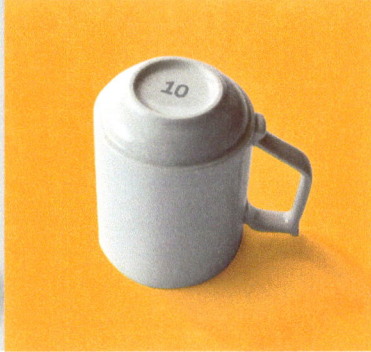
Dial	**Speedometer**
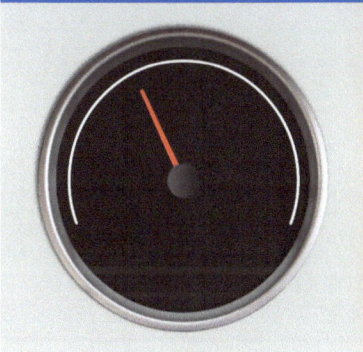	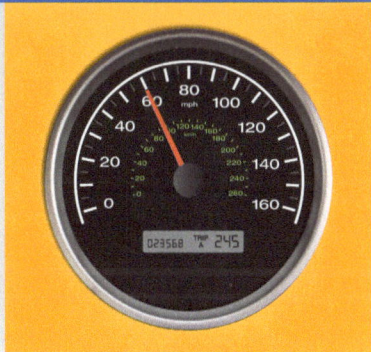

Note from author...

Thank you for taking the time to read this book. I hope you find that I am not trying to sell you a diet or a set of dishes. I am trying to sell you the idea that you can easily implement today and reap the benefits in your health and well-being tomorrow.

My ultimate goal is to change the world of eating so that we can go anywhere and get a Rightsized meal every time. In a restaurant, we should be able to order the Rightsized portion for us. When our children go to a cafeteria, they should be able to select the meal by the size that's right for them. Stores, restaurants, dish manufacturers, food manufacturers, and cafeterias, could implement small changes that would have a profound positive impact on our nation's health. I am working passionately to make this our reality.

I wish you great success on your journey to the optimal you. I encourage you to give the Dish Diet a try. I truly believe that the small steps described in my book will help lead you to your desired destination.

Danuta Highet

P.S. I welcome your feedback from your journey to the Rightsized you. Please share your thoughts. It will help me improve this book and my products.

Dish Diet
P.O. Box 910
New Smyrna Beach, FL 32170

Appendix

Tips for easy to implement incremental changes:

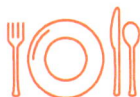

Food and Eating

- Cook smaller quantities, using smaller pots, and eliminate leftovers. Food tastes better when it's fresh anyway and you'll remove the temptation to eat more than you need. If you choose to cook larger quantities to save time, put the leftovers in the refrigerator before you sit down to eat. Freeze these in your Dish Diet Size containers so all you need to do is defrost, heat, and eat.

- Order food online if you can. You will be less tempted to purchase items that are harder to resist when you see them in person.

- Fresh meals that are sent to your home are one-size-fits-all; you can order less often and split the portions for lunches or another meal.

- Do not eat when you are absolutely famished. Have a carrot stick and wait 10-15 minutes.

- Your body has a daily cycle. Work with your metabolism's daily cycles, not against them. Your metabolism runs at high speed during the day. At night it slows down, so eating big meals late at night will cause you to gain more weight and may result in heartburn and indigestion. If you have to have something at night, make it a small snack. (And a smaller snack next time, and smaller...)

- If you order pizza, ask for the small and ask them to double slice it (or you can double slice it at home).

- Today's small used to be large. What used to be small is now called "individual" in many places.

Kitchen

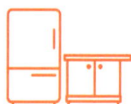

- Remove dishes that are bigger than your size from your cabinets.

- Rearrange your cabinets and refrigerators. It costs you nothing but a little bit of time. Take a tip from the supermarkets – put what you should be eating at eye level.

- Hide your vices from your eyes.

- Hide your cookbooks from the counter-top and put nice photos of delicious fresh vegetables.

- Change your utensils. Smaller spoons/forks means taking more bites. The demitasse spoon may be your future dinner spoon.

- The baking-ware has also been up-sized. Shrink your baking-ware and cut the serving pieces smaller.

Living Space

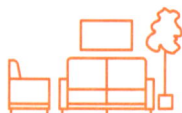

- Go through your house and remove objects that make you think of eating. Instead, choose images that make you want to move more like: nature, outdoor activities, happy active family photos, or calming abstracts.

- Replace what triggers your thoughts of food with thoughts of activity.

- Out of sight, out of mind. Remember this as you redesign your surroundings.

- Where your candy dish stood before, put a weight for training and lifting while you have a free moment.

- Remove every chocolates plate and replace it with a book about healthy living.

- Put a jump rope and weights in the TV room. Use them during shows or commercials.

- Put a water bottle next to your TV chair.

Activities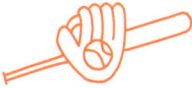

- Stop playing video games that have food in them.

- Stop watching cooking shows if you find that you are thinking about food right after watching.

- Fast forward through commercials or record shows and movies without commercials. Battle the bulge with the mute button.

- The Food Channel and cooking shows will not help you lose weight. They display huge portions.

- If your commute takes you past a lot of restaurants and billboards with food ads, change your route. A relaxing drive through the countryside may add a couple of minutes to your commute, but you will get home more relaxed and not as hungry. Drive by tennis courts, golf courses, or gyms instead.

Food Shopping

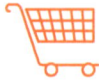

- Do not grocery shop when you are hungry. Take a shopping list, and stick to it. Shop right after dinner; moving around will help digestion.

- Repackage bulk foods into smaller, opaque containers. Just label them so you know what's inside.

- Remove labels (if possible) that make bad things look appetizing. You can put your own labels on them like: "Hip booster," "Waist expander," "X-Large guaranteed."

- Sodas and fruit juices have a high CDM. The more sugar you consume, the less you taste it. A way to help wean yourself off of the sweet drinks is to gradually cut the sugar content by diluting the drink with small amounts of water or club soda.

- Don't buy junk food but if you must, hide it – preferably behind your exercise equipment.

Friends, Family, and Pets

- Stay away from buffets. Buffets only tempt you into trying everything. If there are 20 different entrees, you will feel compelled to try them all. Then you have to try the different soups and salads and desserts. By the time you finish "taste-testing," you will have eaten enough food for five people.

- With friends, sit so that chips and snacks are out of reach. Keep a glass of water next to your hand at all times.

- In a restaurant order an appetizer that fits on your Dish Size Plate. Limit yourself to what fits and make it last.

- Eat slowly. Enjoy every morsel of food. Identify the flavors and the ingredients. Feel the texture, chew tiny pieces, and enjoy each one. If you are not enjoying it, why are you eating it?

- "Slow-pace" your slowest friends. Eat one chip for every 10 chips they eat.

- Can't get a smaller plate or bowl, think camouflage. Fill up your dish with low CDM foods to cover the "white space". Decorate your outer plate area with lettuce and put the entree in the center.

- Restaurants are coming out with new "Bite Size" desserts. These are still high-calorie, high Caloric Density Mark foods.

- Help Fido. If your pet has weight issues talk to your vet; reducing portions gradually for your pets will help optimize their health.

- If you have to have foods you crave at home, keep them out of sight and out of reach. Put them in closed containers that you can't see through.

- Put healthier, lower CDM foods in places that are easier to reach.

References

1   US Patent: US20160117950A1
     "Incrementally-sized standard-sized eating-ware
     system for weight management"

     and

     US Patent: US20090035734A1
     "Incrementally-sized dishware system and method of
     using same for weight management"

2   http://en.wikipedia.org

3-6 http://www.brainyquote.com

7   Brian Wansink. *Mindless Eating: Why We Eat More
     Than We Think.* Bantam, 2007. page 30.

8-13 http://www.brainyquote.com

www.ingramcontent.com/pod-product-compliance
Lightning Source LLC
Chambersburg PA
CBHW041218270326
41931CB00001B/19